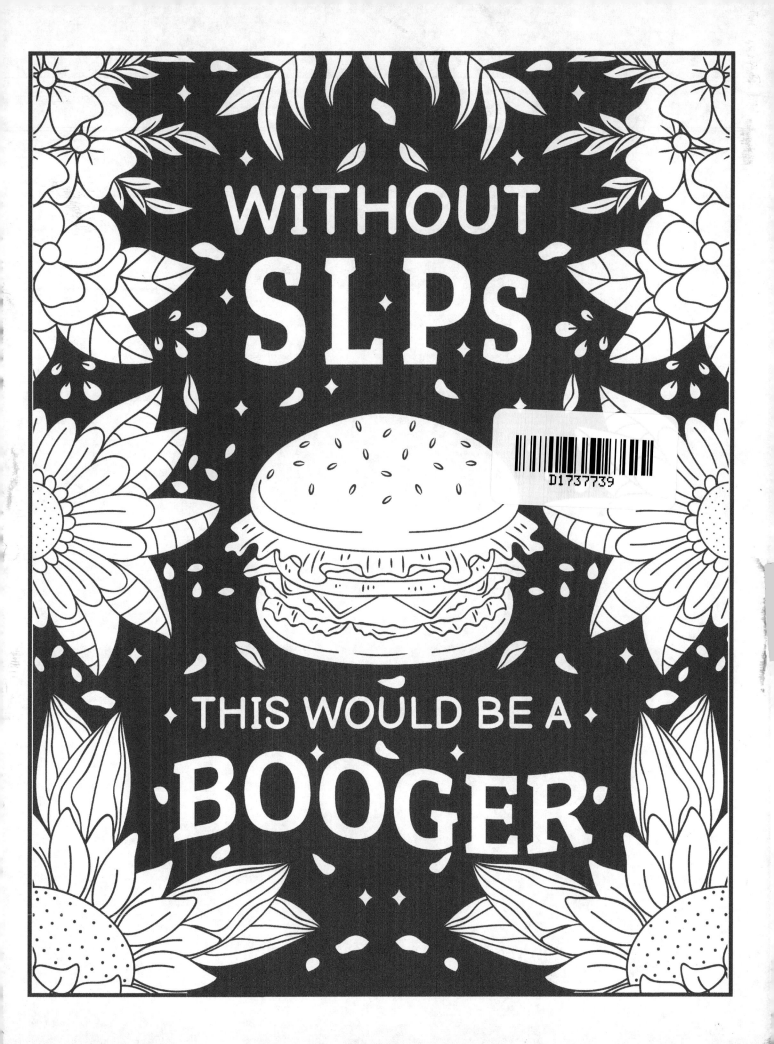

Published by Abinash Mutuwa Publishing

COLOR TEST PAGE

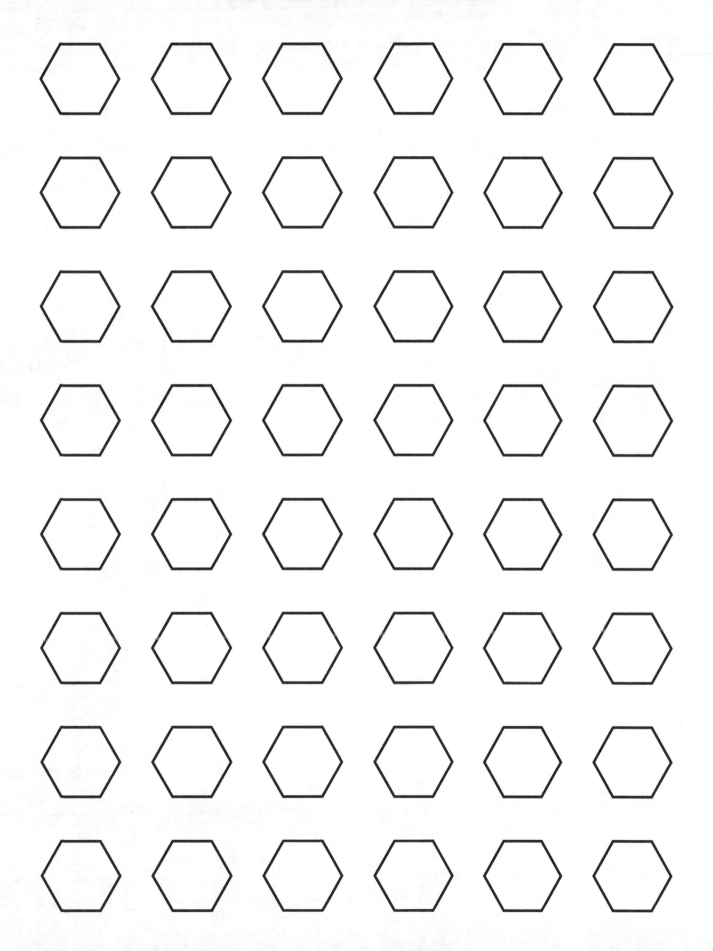

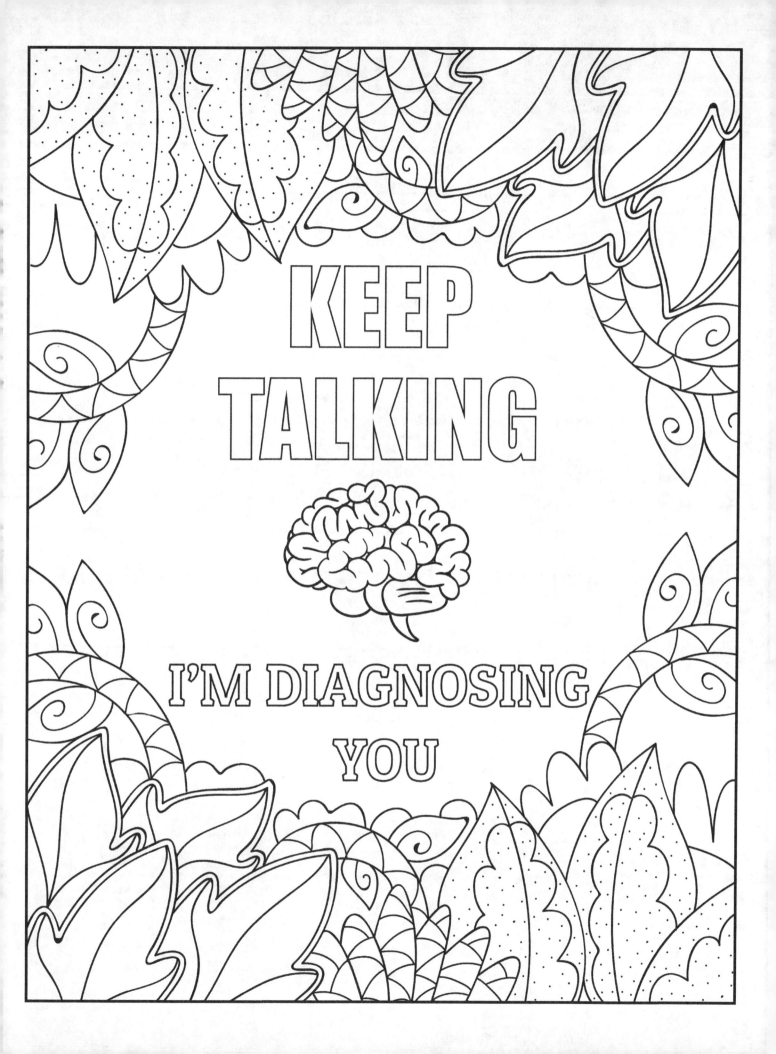

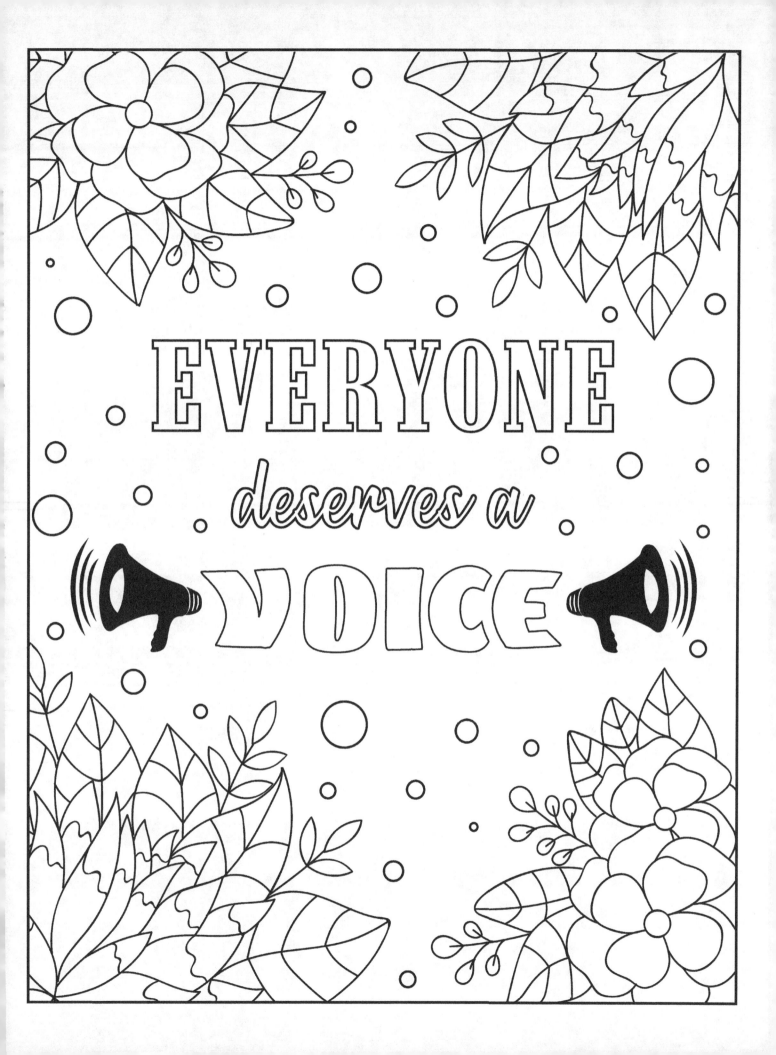

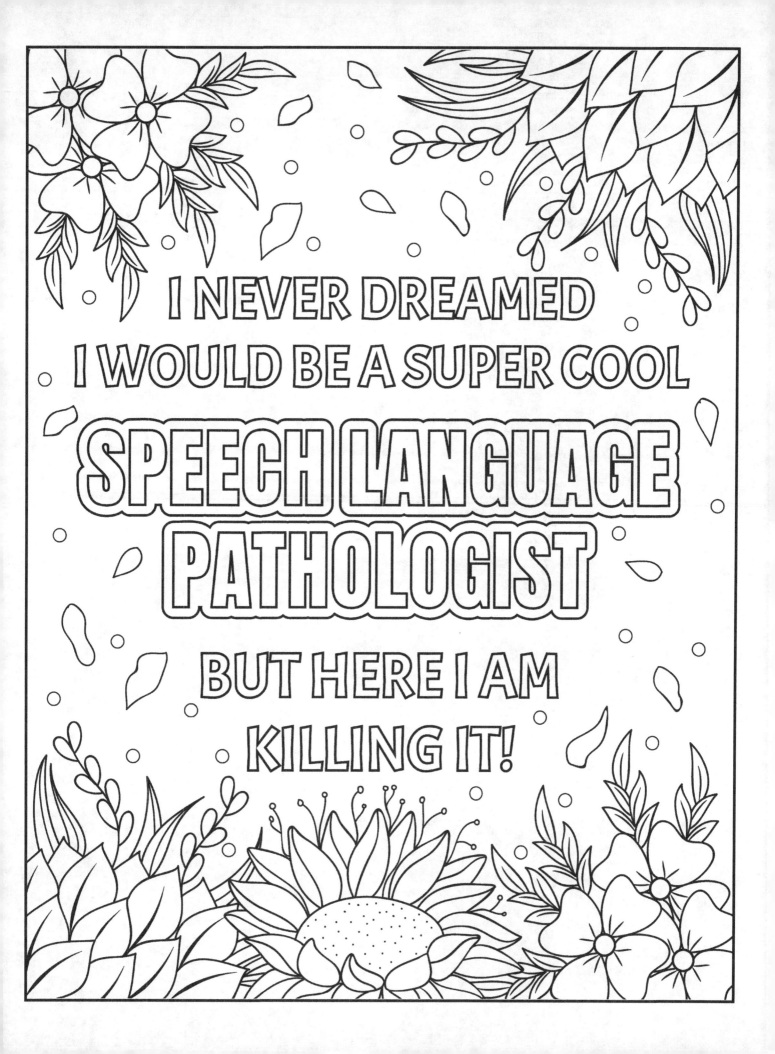

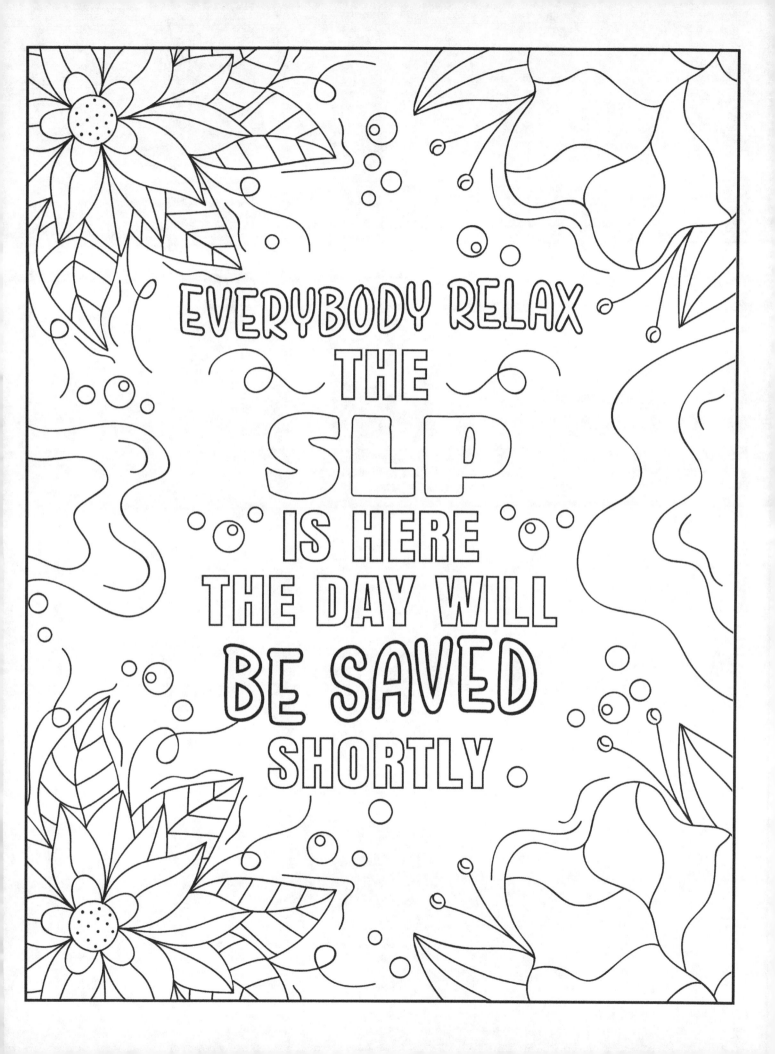

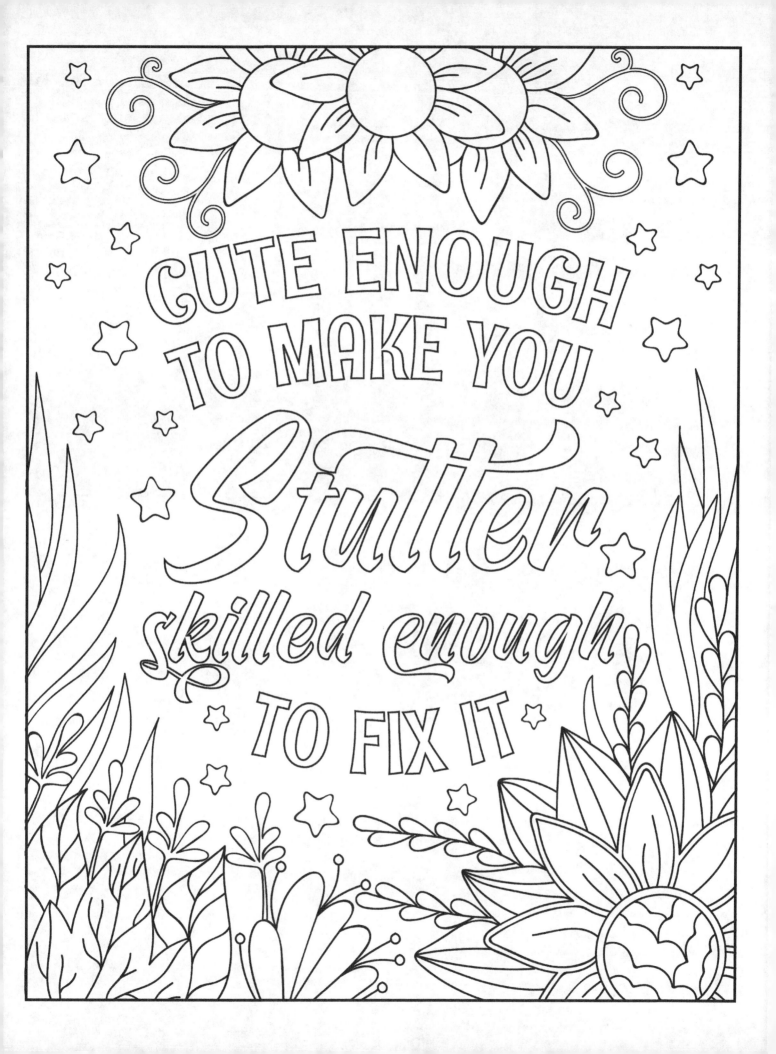

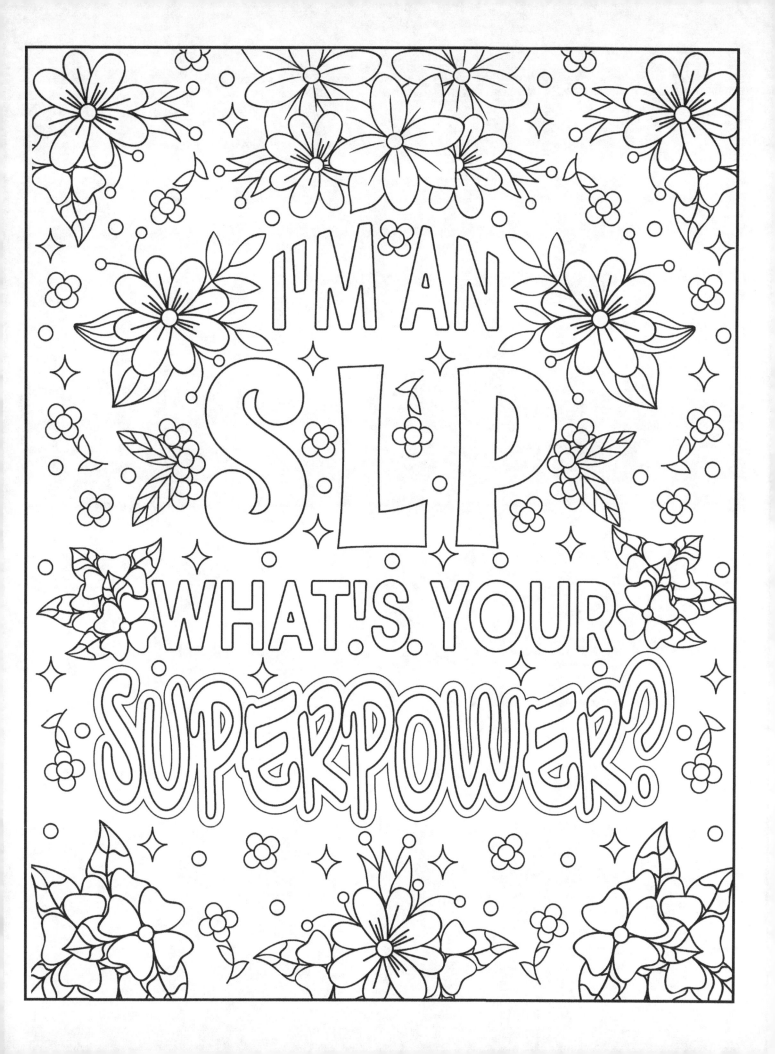

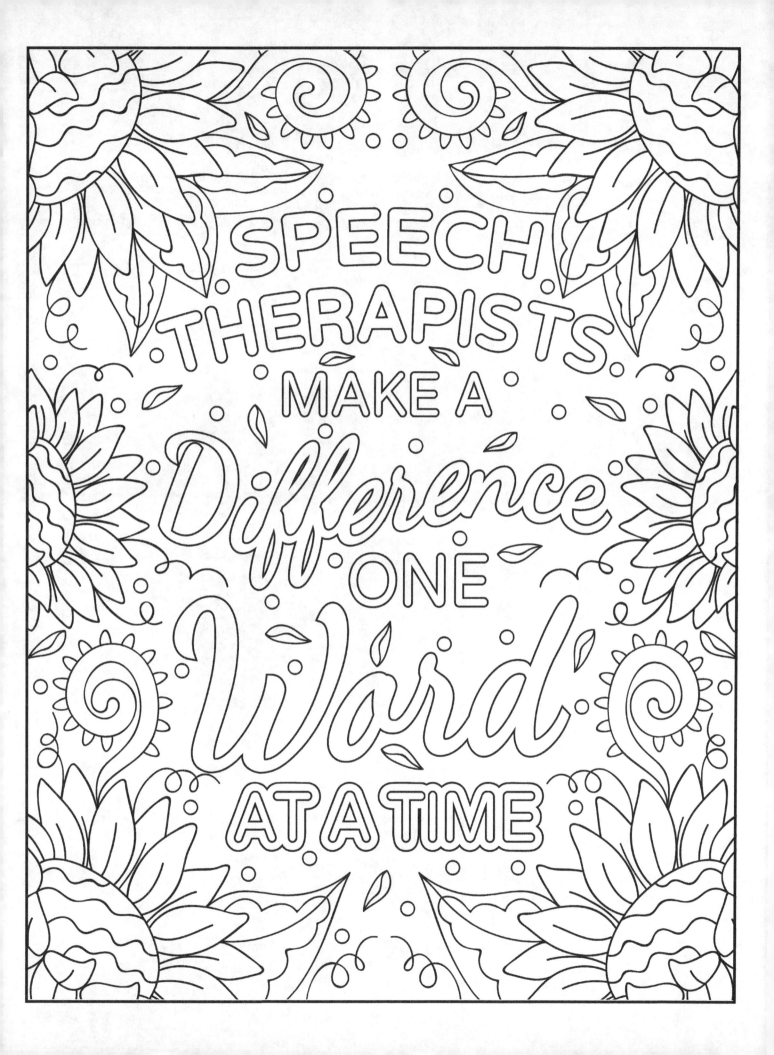

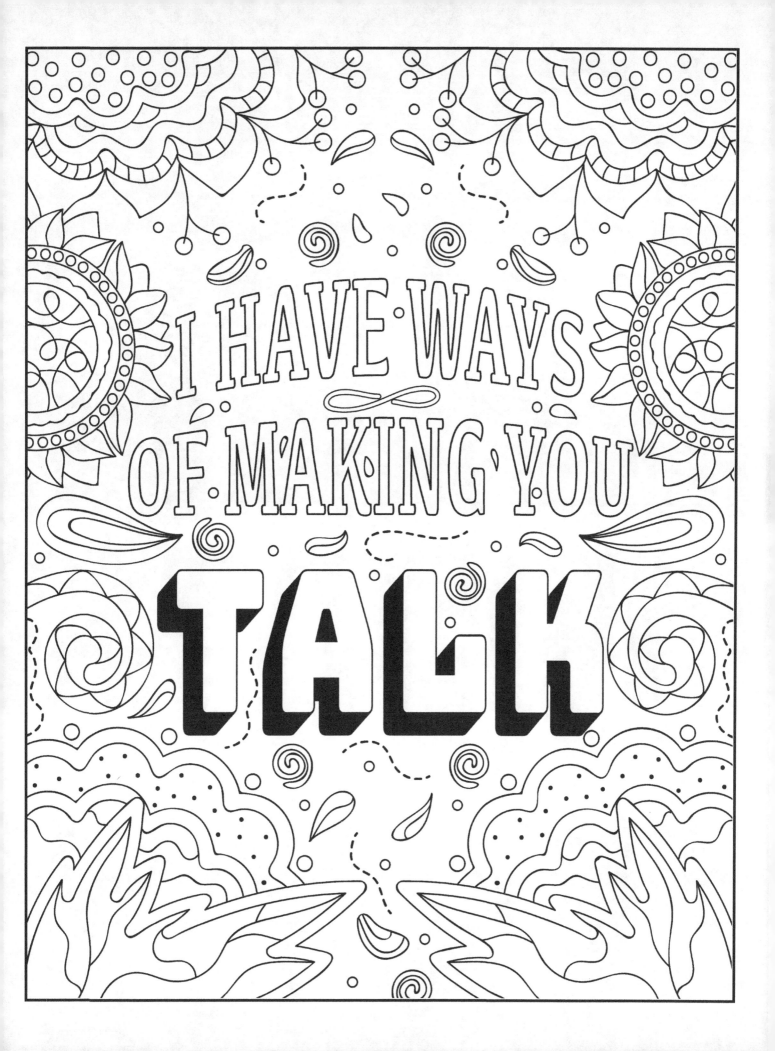

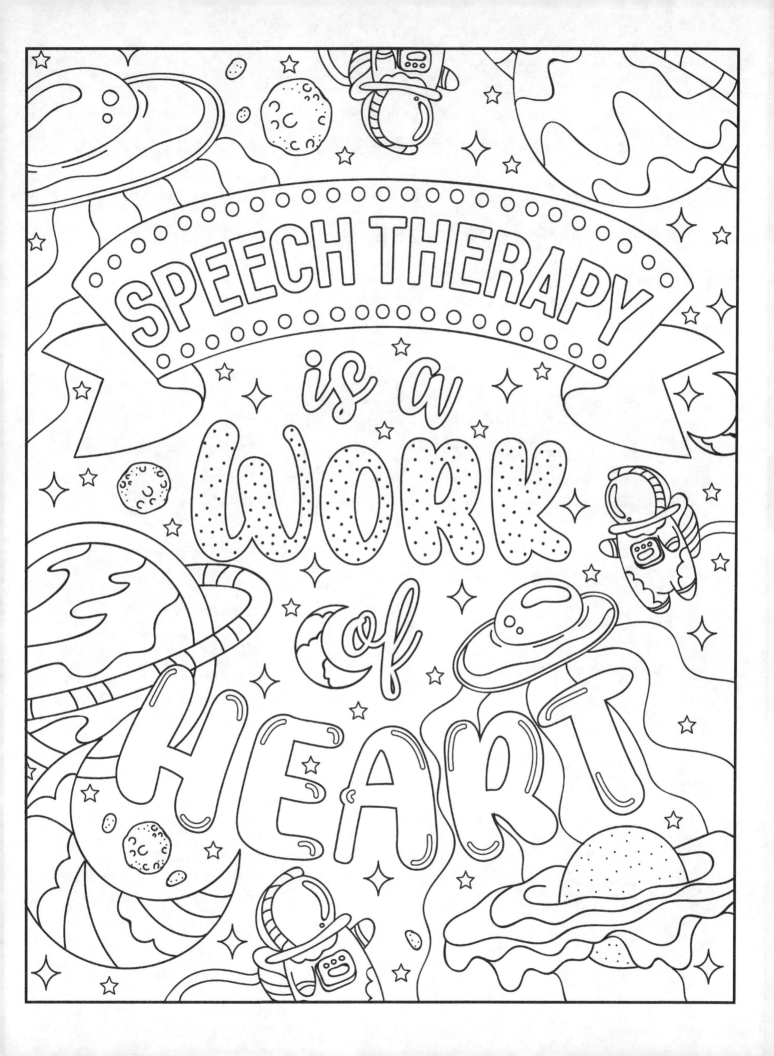

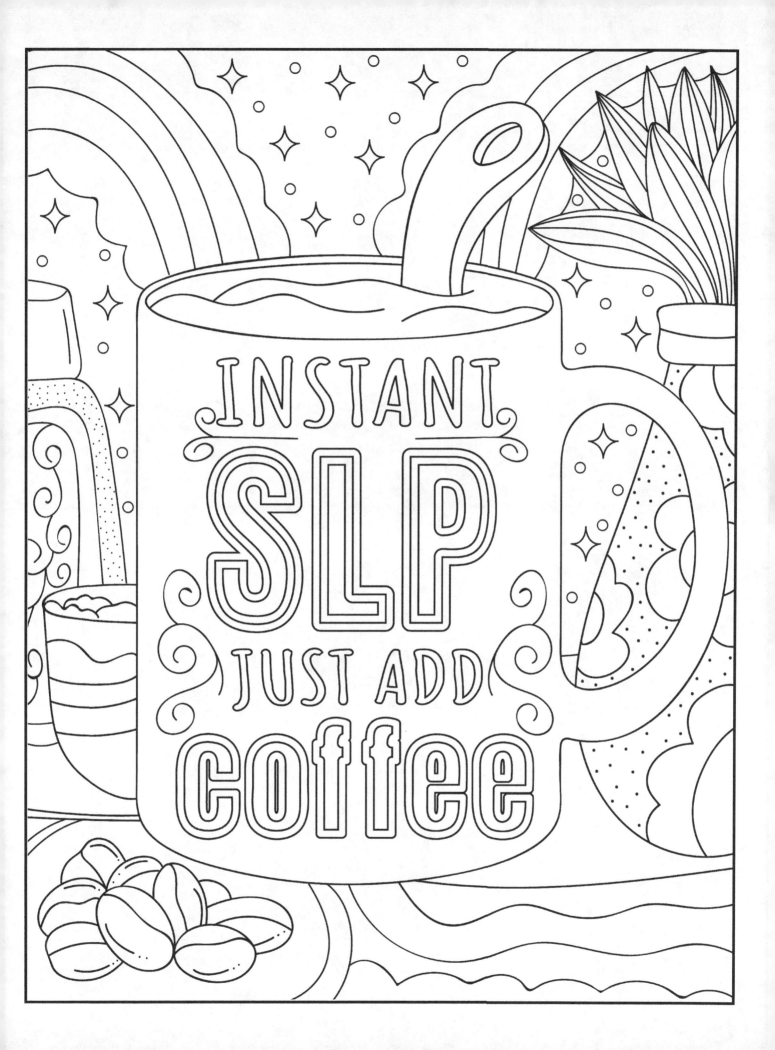

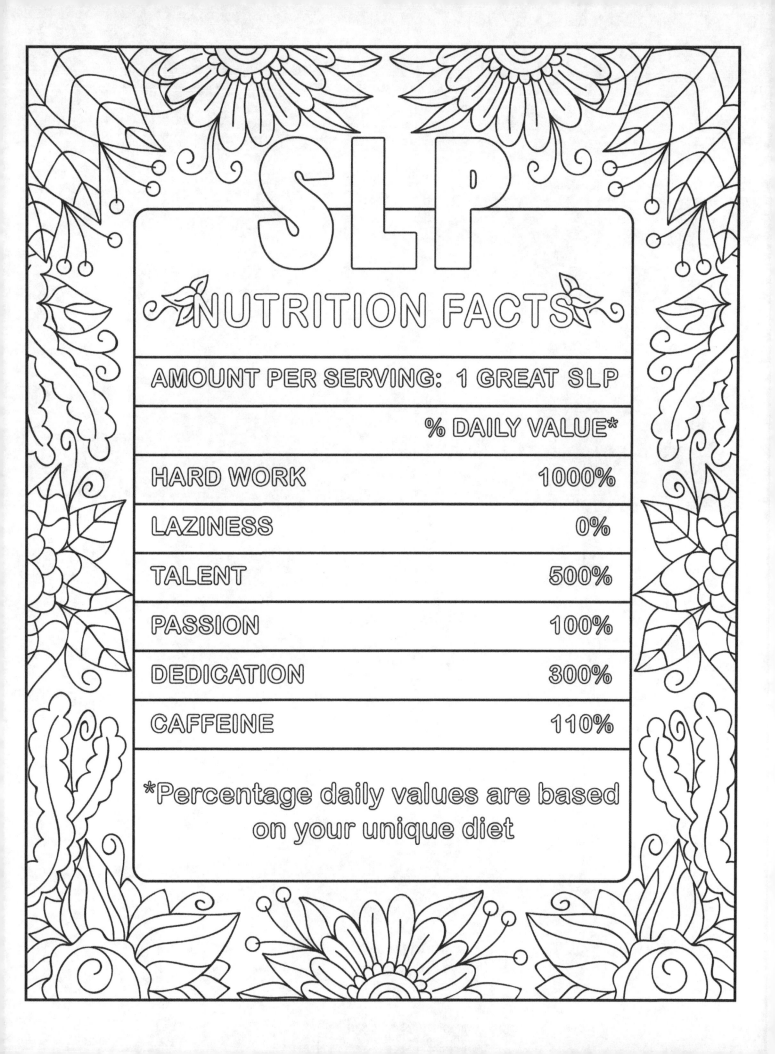

SLP

NUTRITION FACTS

AMOUNT PER SERVING: 1 GREAT SLP

% DAILY VALUE*

HARD WORK	1000%
LAZINESS	0%
TALENT	500%
PASSION	100%
DEDICATION	300%
CAFFEINE	110%

*Percentage daily values are based on your unique diet

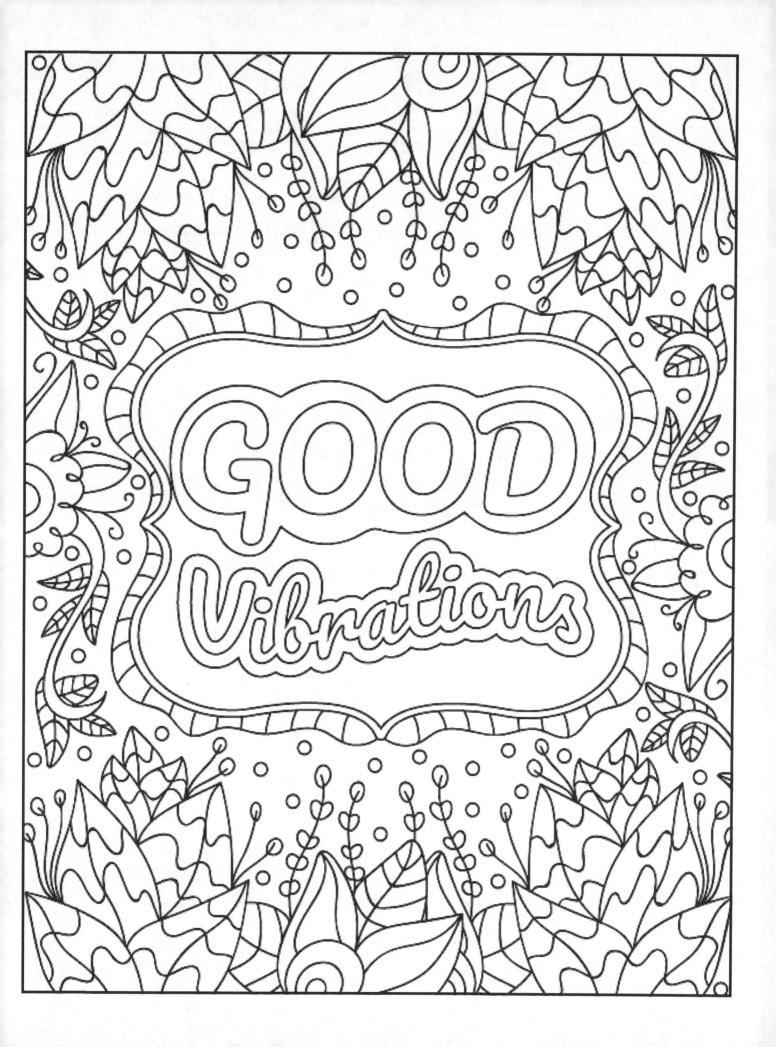

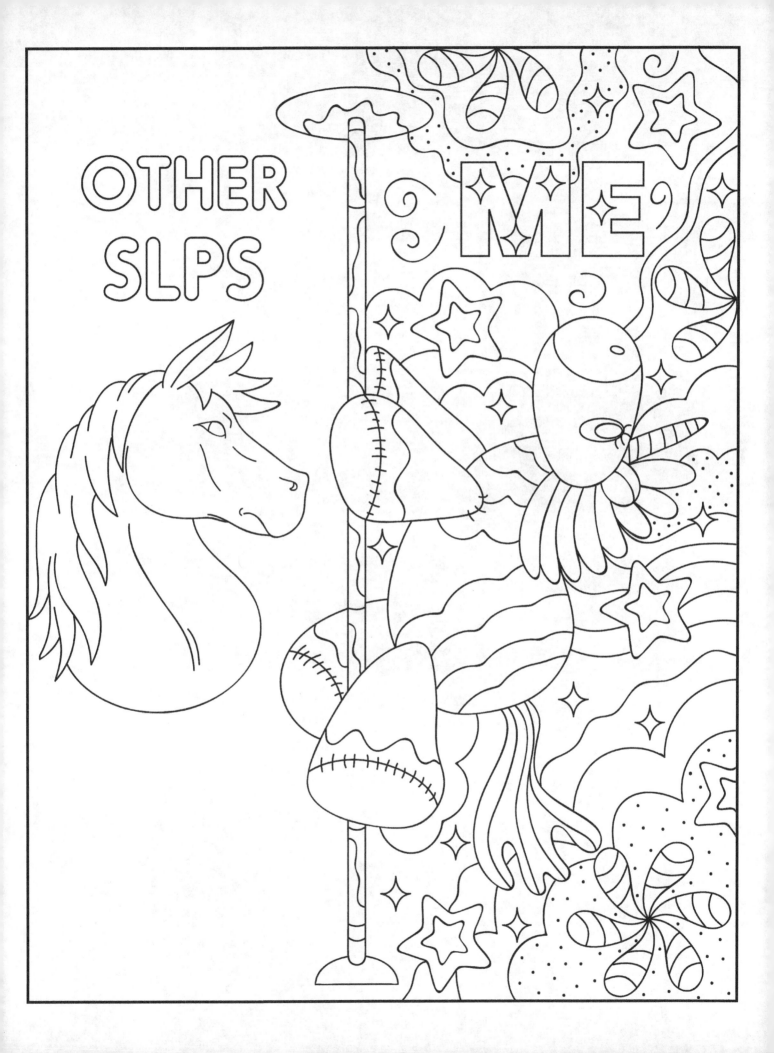

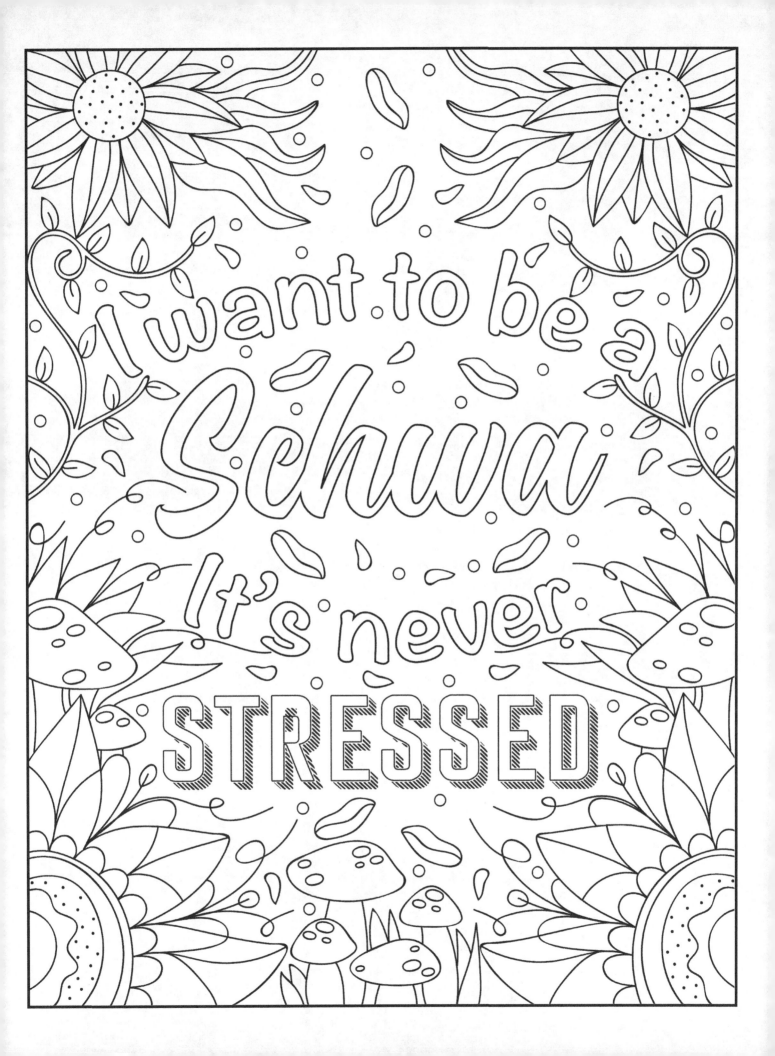

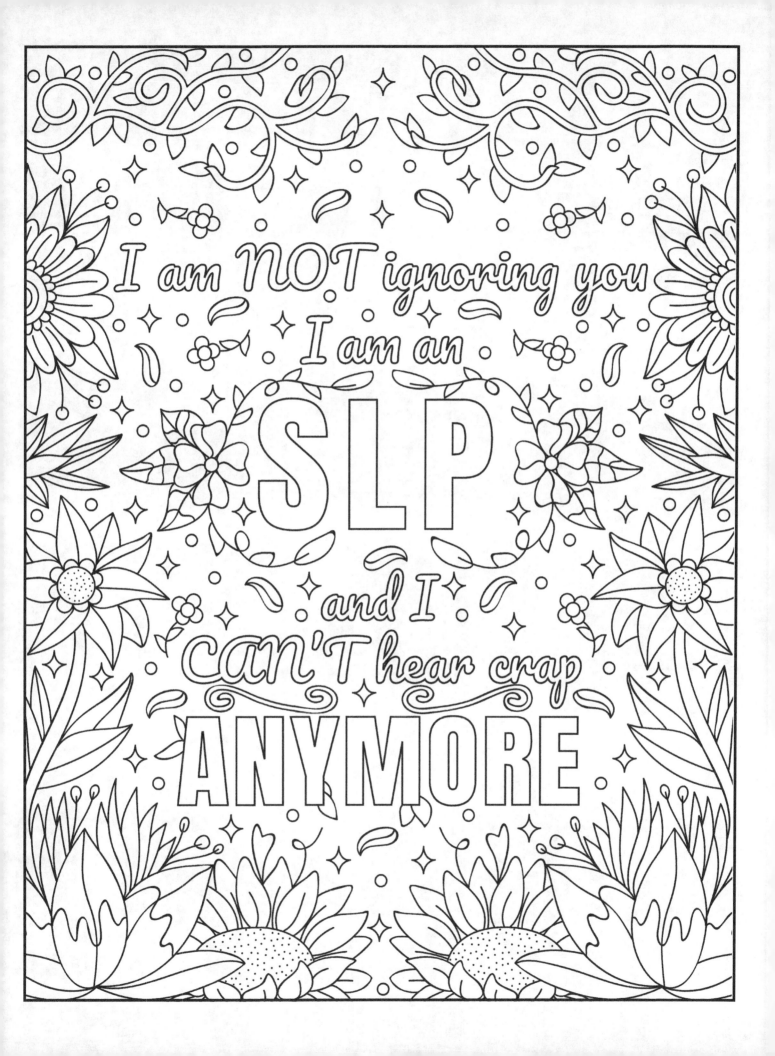

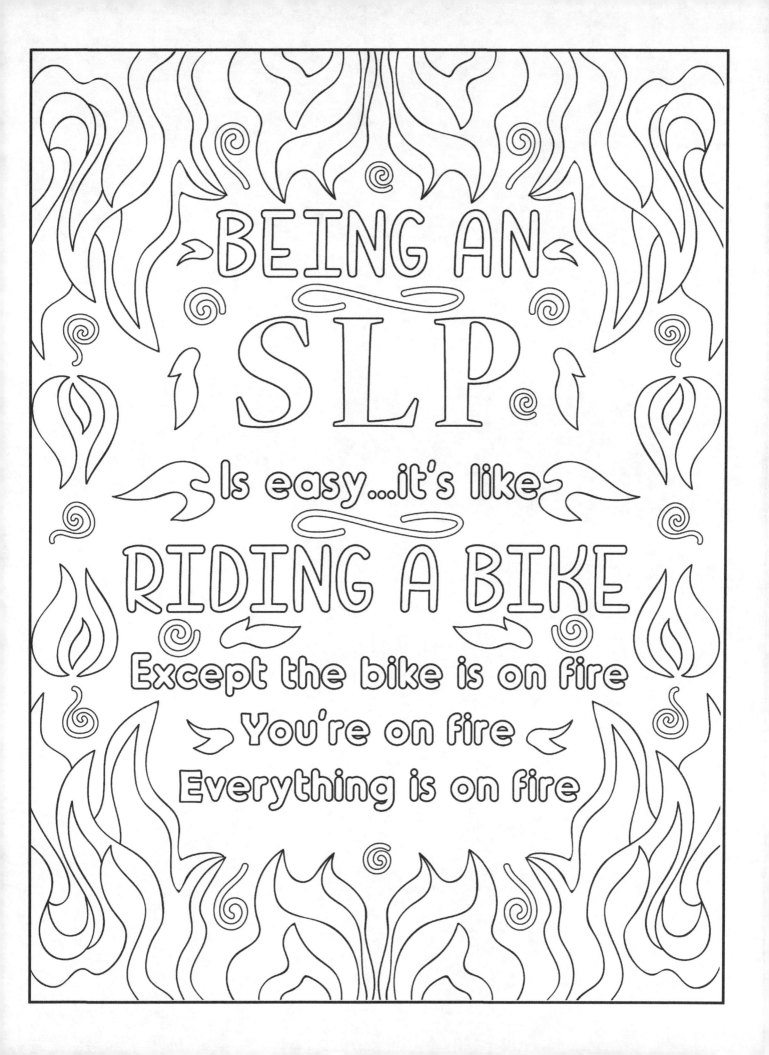

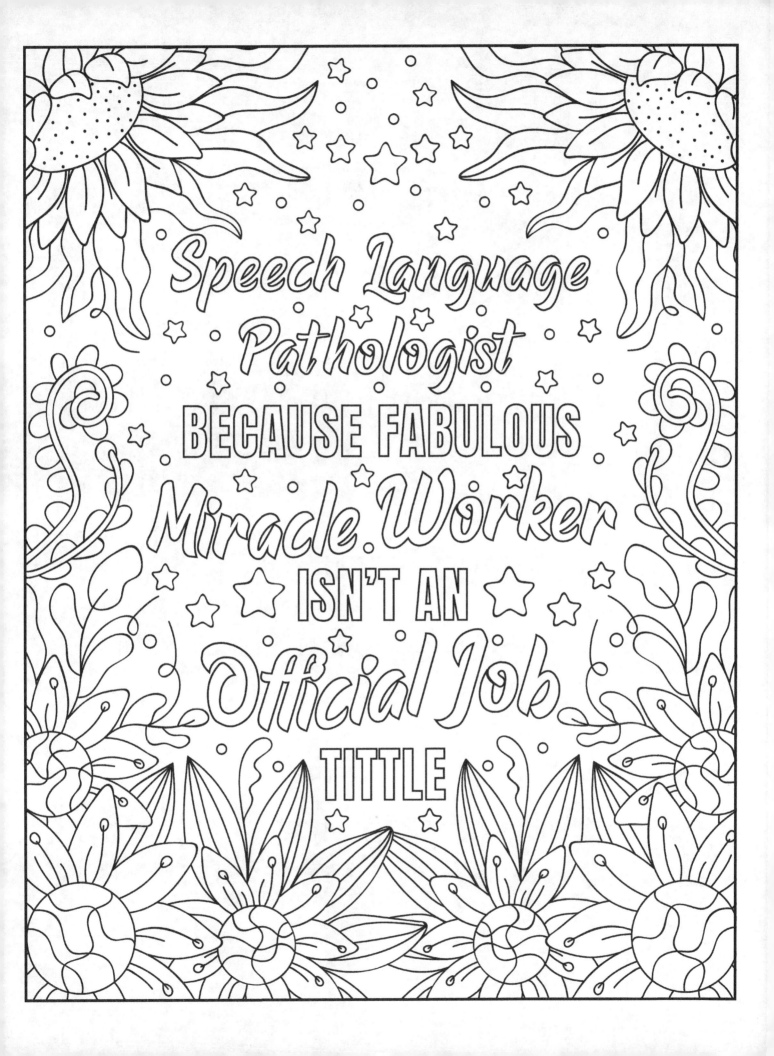

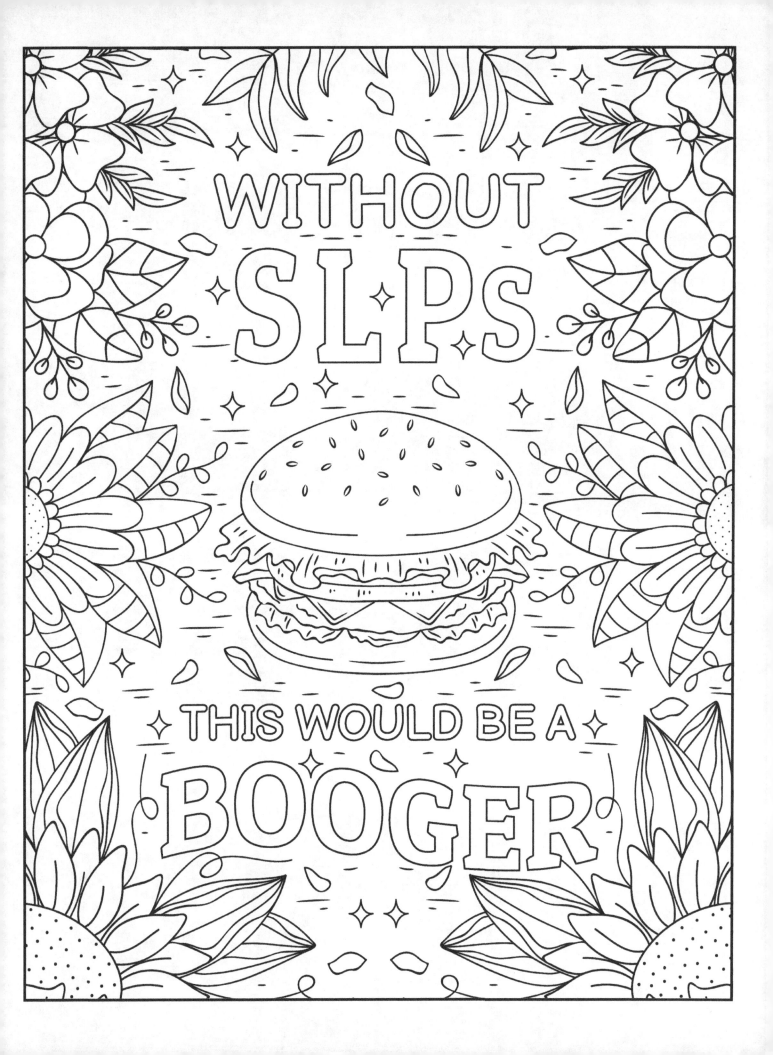

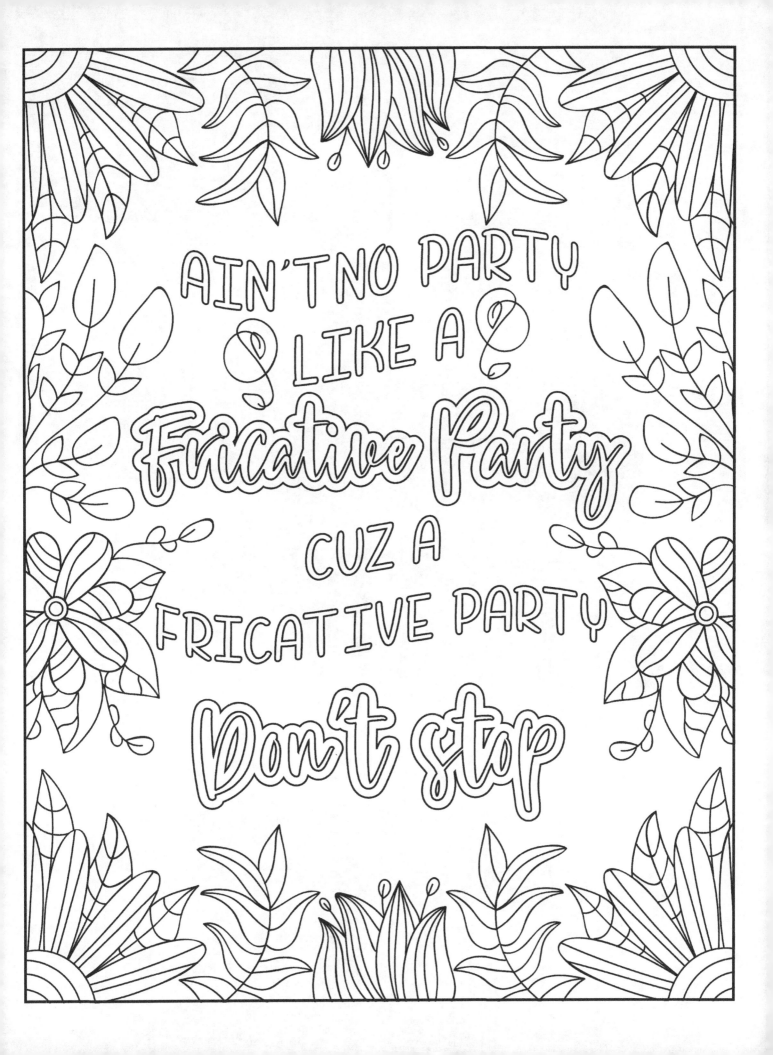

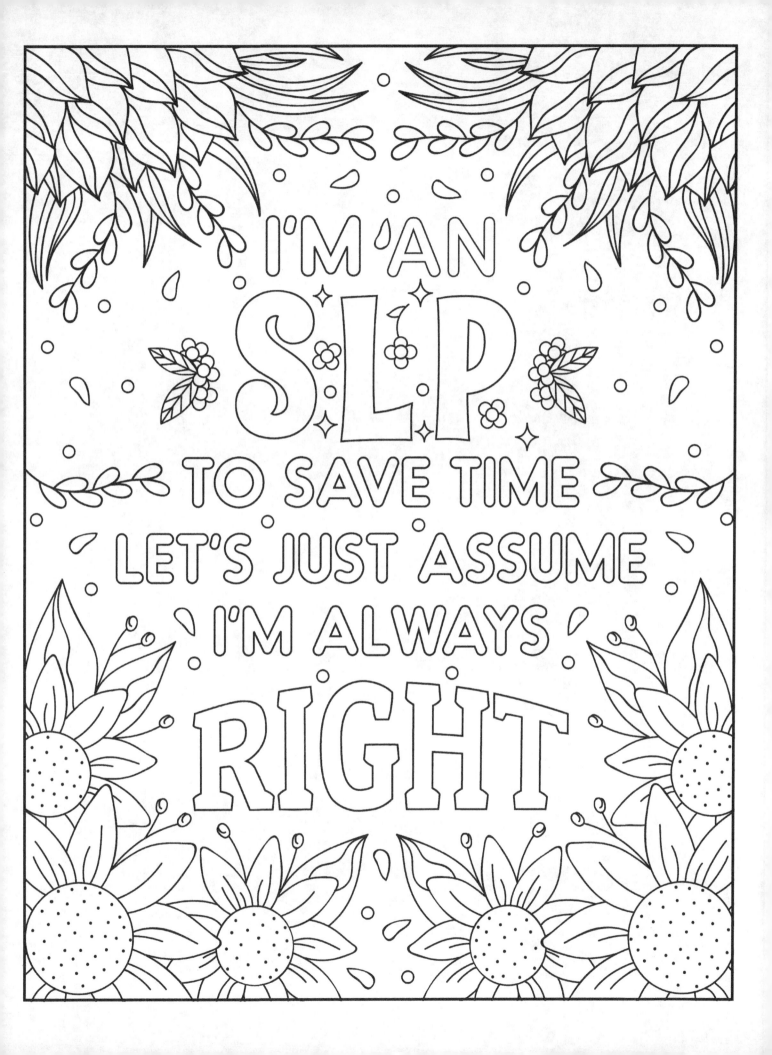

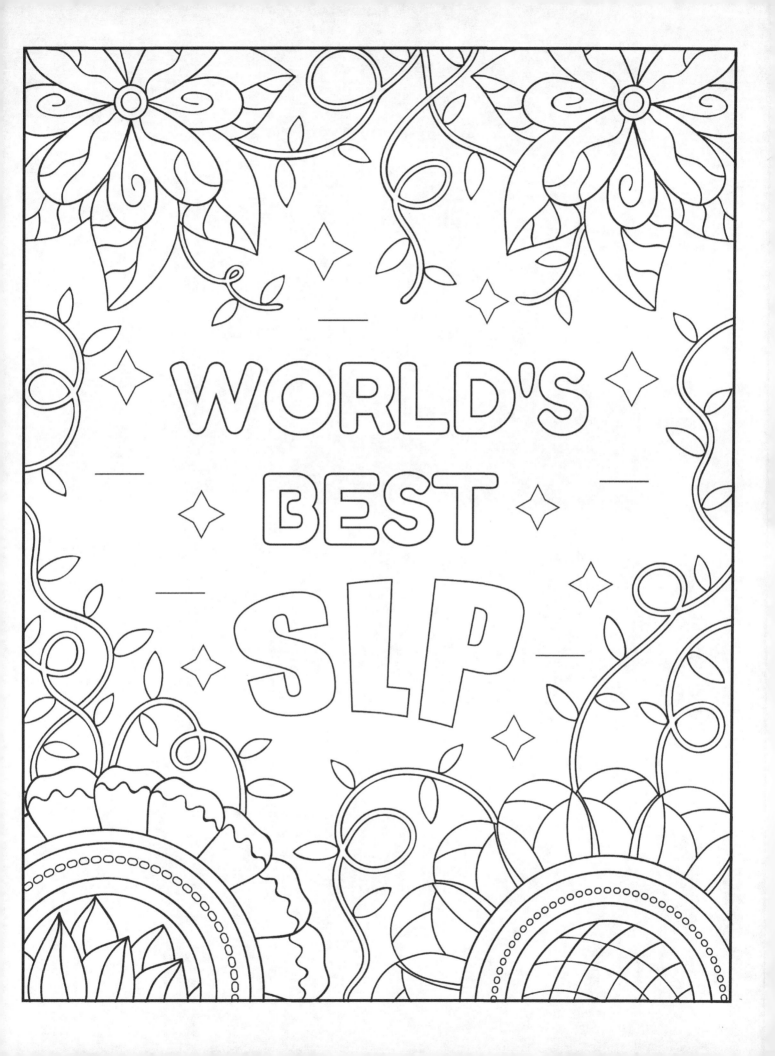

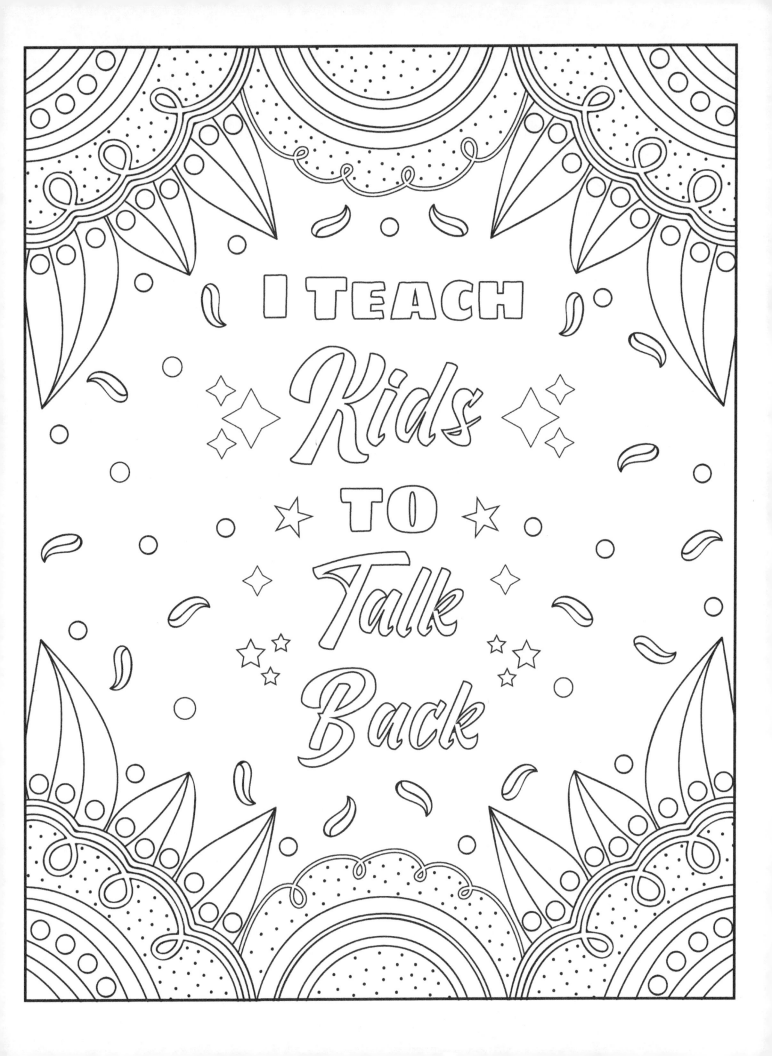

Made in the USA
Las Vegas, NV
04 November 2024